KRATOM

*Everything You Need to Know About Kratom
(Powder, Extract, Capsules, Herbal Supplement)
for Pain Management: Its Uses, Benefits, Possible
Side Effects, Dosage and Interactions*

Table of Content

Introduction

In recent years, an herb known as Kratom has gained popularity as an alternative medicine for pain relief in the West. It is considered to be beneficial for both physical and mental health.

Students and busy people who need more concentration and energy are taking it to cope with the demands of the present age. Those who suffer from various physical ailments have started using it to get relief from pain. Besides this, people plagued by mental disorders resort to this wonderful plant to overcome, brain fog, stress, anxiety, and depression.

However, this miracle cure is not new, instead it has a long-standing history. It has been used since ancient times as a part of folk medicine in the East.

Kratom, officially known as Mitragyna Speciosa, is a plant found mainly in Indonesia, Thailand, Malaysia, and Myanmar. It is related to the coffee plant. It has a euphoric effect like opiates. Many people claim that it is very useful.

It increases energy levels and alertness. Makes people more comfortable in society and able to talk with ease. Moreover, it gives them the capacity to perform tedious tasks.

It is a natural herbal supplement cure for pain relief, anxiety, depression, cancer, hangover, addiction, and arthritis.

Let us learn how to use it safely in the form of powder, capsules, or extract and benefit from it.

Chapter I

What is Kratom

Kratom, or Mitragyna Speciosa, is a tropical evergreen that belongs to Southeast Asia. Generally, it is found growing wild in southern and central Thailand, Indonesia, Malaysia, Myanmar, and other places in the Pacific Rim. Kratom is also known as biak, ketum, kakum, thom, and thang.

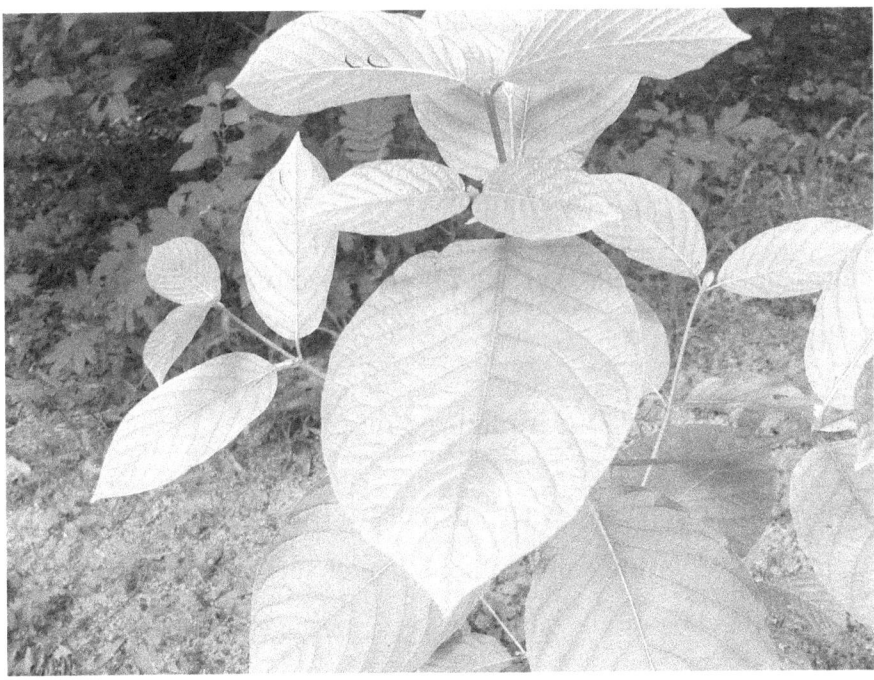

It grows to a height of 42 feet or 13 meters and has deep yellow colored flowers that hang in clusters. There are many uses of Kratom in folk medicine. The broad green leaves of the plant are plucked, dried under the sun, and brewed to be consumed in the form of tea. Otherwise, they are pulverized and then swallowed with some water.

Kratom has been gaining popularity all over the world since the 21st century. It is considered to be an invaluable asset for physical and mental health. Besides this, it also has recreational value for people who use it as a stimulant or as a sedative-narcotic on the basis of the dose consumed.

In Southeast Asia, Mitragyna Speciosa leaves are chewed fresh, brewed and taken as a tea with lemon and honey, or smoked to help day laborers combat fatigue.

In Malaysia and Thailand Kratom is embedded so deeply in the culture of the region that the people hardly consider it to be a drug.

A Brief History of This Amazing Plant

Kratom has been used since ancient times in the native growing areas to cure various ailments. Its leaves were used to make the pains and aches numb, soothe fevers, manage diabetes, alleviate addiction, and treat diarrhea. They were applied in the form of poultices on wounds and spread on the stomach to drive the worms out.

They were popularly used to get energy just like coca, which is used for the same purpose in the Andes. The peasant workers in Thailand used to chew the leaves around ten times a day when they worked in the hot sun.

In Malaysia, it has been used since the early years of the 19th century as a sedative in place of opium.

There was a growing enthusiasm for the medical potential of Kratom, so in 1921 mitragynine, an active constituent of Kratom, was isolated. It was tested on human beings in 1932. The results showed that it had a stimulant effect on the nervous system just like cocaine.

In 1930, two botanists, Mohammed Haniff and I.H. Burkill, reported in Cambridge Journal that throughout the 19th century Kratom was effectively used by opiate users as a means of harm reduction.

By the early years of the 1940s, the revenue of the Thailand government that accrued from the opium tax declined massively. The addicts started using Kratom, which was an unregulated drug, for managing the withdrawal symptoms. In August of 1943, an act was promulgated known as Kratom Act. It forbade the people from cultivating Kratom and ordered that all the existing specimens should be destroyed.

Scientific interest in Kratom grew in other places. During the 1960s scientists isolated over 20 alkaloids. Kratom's second basic active compound 7-hydroxymitragynine was identified in 1994. The next year, mitragynine's first synthesis was done.

The public became aware of Kratom in the early years of the 2000s through online message boards.

However, in 2005 Australia scheduled mitragynine and M. speciosa. It could not be sold or possessed without a license.

In Thailand, arrests in connection with the Kratom Act increased between the years 2005 to 2009. In fact, in 2012, the locals resisted when hundreds of Kratom trees that were growing wild in one protected forest area of Satun Province were ordered to be destroyed.

Many campaigns and advocacy groups have come up in the US, such as the Botanical Education Alliance, United Kratom Association, and American Kratom Association, to safeguard the legality of Kratom. As a result of their efforts, the DEA had to withdraw a proposal to put Kratom on the list of controlled substances in August 2016.

Current Use

In the present, people's interest in the plant is continuously growing. A survey shows that out of 6150 users of Kratom, 9%

use it for withdrawal symptoms of opium, 14% to overcome anxiety, and 51% to reduce pain.

Despite being criminalized and having a social stigma associated with it, Kratom continues to be used in Thailand. When 1000 teenagers were surveyed it was found that 94% of them used Kratom.

In 2014, it was found to be among the topmost 20 drugs in Hungary.

Chemical Constitution of Kratom

Kratom contains indole alkaloids - $C_{23}H_{30}N_2O_4$ mitragynine or methoxy-corynantheidine, $C_{23}H_{30}N_2O_5$ 7-hydroxymitragynine, and other phytochemicals.

Mitragynine is similar to ergine (LSA) and psilocybin because of its structure (4-substituted). Earlier, it was considered the basic active compound. But recently, it has become known that 7-hydroxymitragynine the terpenoid is more potent (46 times) and has a higher oral bioavailability as well as barrier penetration of the blood-brain.

The mechanism involved in the stimulant effect of Kratom is not clear. Both the compounds interact with opioid receptors, so there are chances of the involvement of another alkaloid.

Kratom is one organic substance that has multiple strains. There are diverse methods for its preparation. Therefore, it has a complex chemical composition which has dynamic effects.

The main alkaloids present in it are mitragynine, speciociliatine, paynanthine, and 7-hydroxymitragynine.

Mitragynine is considered to be the basic active alkaloid but Dr. Z. Hassan and others suggest that it could be less powerful than 7-HMG which is less abundant.

Chapter II

Varieties of Kratom

The types of Kratom are divided on the basis of their colors. This classification is done on the basis of the leaf's vein and stem color. The colors determine the effect that a leaf has on the body and mind.

Different colors have different chemical compositions and therefore have different effects. Their effects also vary from one vendor to another. Various colored strains of Kratom thrive under different conditions. Different kinds of Kratom are known as strains.

Red Vein

- This is the most popular strain available in the market. It is very good for beginners as it produces a pleasant calming effect. It grants mental peace and makes you feel optimistic. It helps to overcome insomnia. It relaxes the muscles and relieves pain. Extracts of red Kratom are used by opiate addicts to stay away from withdrawal symptoms.
- There are a number of differences between the properties and effects of various red veins. Some strains like Red

Borneo and Red Thai have sedative effects while Red Sumatra brings about an elevation of mood.

- The effects also vary according to the dose. Small doses of red vein have a stimulating influence. Overall the strains of red vein are used for promoting tranquility and peace.

White Vein

- This type of Kratom vein is known to be a mood enhancer and stimulant. People take it instead of caffeine for concentration, cheerfulness, and alertness. They also take it for increased stamina and motivation when they have to work for long hours.
- This variety of Kratom is suitable for people who feel exhausted or go through gloomy periods. However, it should not be taken towards the end of the day because the person may have restless sleep.
- Usually, white vein and red vein powders are mixed and taken to boost energy in a balanced way.

Green Vein

- It has an effect which is in between that of the white and red veins. It gives a mild boost of energy and can brighten up a person's mood.

- It helps to enhance focus and alertness. It does not cause drowsiness like the other analgesics and can be used to relieve pain.
- Green vein can be combined with the other two veins to avoid the red vein's excessive anesthesia and the white vein's overstimulation.
- Green vein has a balanced functioning and is used to remove social fears. It makes a person more talkative, cheerful, and friendly.

Most of the varieties are named after their place of origin such as Bali and Indo Kratoms which originated in Indonesia, Malay Kratom from Malaysia, Thai Kratom from Thailand, and Borneo Kratom from Borneo.

Types of Kratom with Their Effects and Doses

Here is a list of various types of Kratom with their effects and doses.

Bali

- It has a euphoric effect. It is like an opiate.
- Dose - 1/2 to 3 tsp

Maeng Da

- It has a stimulating and energizing effect. Gives relief from pain.
- Dose - 1/2 to 3 tsp

Thai Red Vein

- It has a euphoric effect. It is like an opiate.
- Dose - 1/2 to 3 tsp

Kali Red Vein

- It has a sedating effect. It is like an opiate.
- Dose - 1/2 to 3 tsp

Red Indo

- It has a sedating effect.
- Dose - 1/2 to 3 tsp

Green Indo

- Gives relief from pain and boosts energy.
- Dose - 1/2 to 3 tsp

Kali Green Vein

- It has a stimulating effect. It also gives relief from pain.
- Dose - 1/2 to 3 tsp

Kali White Vein

- More euphoric effect.
- Dose - 1/2 to 3 tsp

Thai White Vein

- More euphoric effect.
- Dose 1/2 to 3 tsp

Indo White Vein

- It has a sedating effect. Gives relief from pain.
- Dose - 1/2 to 3 tsp

Super Indo

- It has a euphoric effect which is lesser than Bali.
- Dose - 1/2 to 3 tsp

Malaysian Super Green

- It has a stimulating effect.
- Dose - 1/2 to 3 tsp

Indo Ultra Enhanced

- Most euphoric among the extracts. Helps to reduce social anxiety.

- Dose - 1 g or less (in case it is mixed with the powdered leaf)

Extract - Gold Reserve

- Powerful extract
- Dose - 1 g or less (in case it is mixed with the powdered leaf)

ISOL-8

- Stimulation similar to caffeine.
- Dose - 1 g or less (in case it is mixed with the powdered leaf)

True Thai - Natural Enhanced

- Dose - 1 g or less (in case it is mixed with the powdered leaf)

White Sumatra - Natural Enhanced

- Dose - 1 g or less (in case it is mixed with the powdered leaf)

Chapter III
Regions of Growth

The Kratom plant is originally from Southeast Asia. Here are some of the main regions where Kratom is grown.

Indonesia

Indonesia is located in the middle of the Indian Ocean and Pacific Ocean. It is the biggest island country in the world and has over 13,000 islands.

Indonesia has a tropical climate. There are only two seasons. From November until March it goes through a wet season. During the remaining months, it has a dry season. There is less precipitation during this time and most of the days are sunny. This type of climate is suitable for the growth of Kratom.

Three types of Kratom are grown in Indonesia; they are red, white, and green vein. They are known as Indo Kratom and are very popular.

The different regions in Indonesia where Kratom is grown are as follows:

Borneo

It is the 3rd largest island in the world. Seventy-three percent of its territory is owned by Indonesia. The strains of Kratom that grow in this area:

- White vein or poor man's maeng da
- Red vein (Bali Kratom)
- Green vein

Sumatra

It is the 6th largest island in the world. The strains of Kratom that are grown here:

- Red vein
- White vein

Riau

Even though it is located near Sumatra the strains that are produced here are quite different from Sumatra's strains. The strains from Riau have a nice aroma and a sweeter taste. These are preferred by people who do not like the bitter taste of Kratom.

The main strains grown here are as follows:

- Red Riau
- Green Riau

Malaysia

Malaysia has an equatorial climate. There are two monsoons. In the southwest, the monsoons start in April and go on till October. In the northeast, they begin in October and go on till February.

The Kratom produced in this region is known as Malay Kratom. It is a unique variety of Kratom. It has long-lasting effects that last for 7 to 8 hours. In some cases, the effects may be felt throughout the day.

Smaller doses have a very euphoric effect and higher doses are soothing and relaxing.

Earlier Thai Kratom used to come from Thailand, but Kratom is banned there. So the Thai variety that is available in the market comes from Indonesia. Maeng da is a popular Thai Kratom. Many people consider it to be the best variety because alkaloids are present in a very high concentration.

Chapter IV

Benefits of Kratom

Kratom is an herb from South East Asia that has become very popular in the West in recent years because of its remarkable benefits. This tropical plant which belongs to the same family as coffee is enchanting students and busy people who need more focus and drive.

But its medicinal qualities have been used since ancient times in the East where it originated. Some of its benefits are discussed here.

Relief from Pain

Kratom contains alkaloids with which it has the capacity to relieve pain like a mild opioid. The good part is that it is not addictive like an opioid. The alkaloids work on the opiate receptors in the nervous system. They help in releasing endorphins and enkephalins which numb the pain receptors of the body.

In this way, Kratom offers relief from pain to the patients of osteoarthritis, osteoporosis, osteomalacia, chronic backache, joint pain, and rheumatoid arthritis.

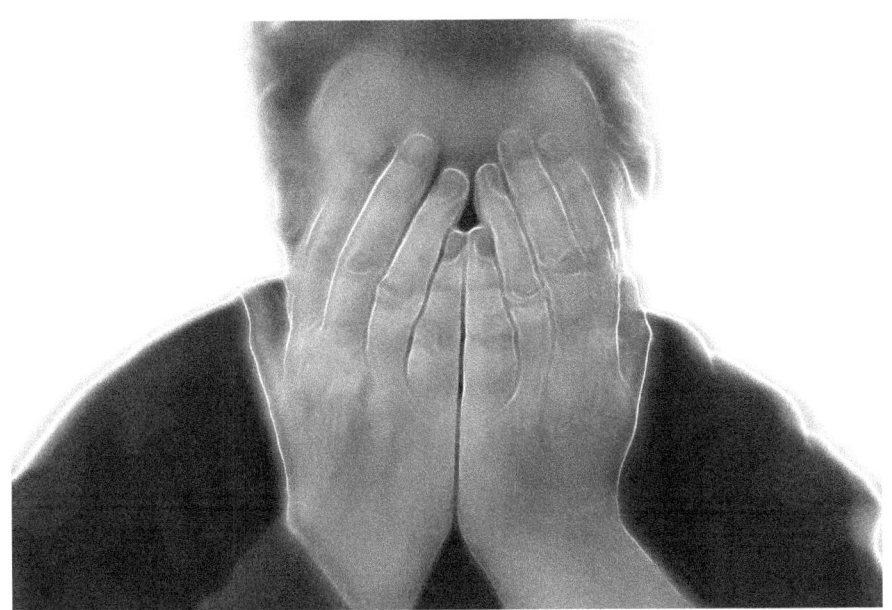

Overcome Addiction

Kratom is not an opiate. However, it activates the opiate receptors present in a person's brain. Kratom bonds with the receptors before an opioid would and thus eases the effect of addiction to some extent. This helps to curb the cravings of the addicts for a drug that they are trying to give up.

Kratom also reduces the symptoms of withdrawal like:

- Cramps
- Nausea
- Vomiting
- Pain
- Sleeplessness
- Anxiety

That is why Kratom has been included in treatments for cases of substance abuse. It has helped addicts to overcome dependency on alcohol and various drugs such as heroin.

Reduce Anxiety, Stress, and Depression

Kratom helps to elevate a person's mood and to soothe the nerves. It is a psychoactive substance and releases serotonin and endorphins that enhance a person's overall mood.

Kratom's calming effect helps to ease tension. This helps to get rid of social anxiety and people feel relaxed and comfortable in such situations. This is the reason why in villages of Southeast Asia people consume Kratom in social gatherings.

It alleviates anxiety symptoms like insomnia, sweating, heart palpitations, muscle cramps, and hyperventilation. Therefore, it is ideal for people who suffer from anxiety, stress, depression, panic attacks, mood swings, and those who work in very demanding jobs.

Quite a few strains of Kratom are stronger than the others. If they are taken in a larger amount, they generate euphoric feelings. This benefit of the herb may be very tempting. But you should find out the amount that you need to get the right effect and not go beyond it.

Increase Your Focus on Studies or Work

You can take Kratom to enhance your productivity. The alkaloids, mitragynine and 7-hydroxymitragynine act on the opiate receptors present in the brain and the periphery and help people to work harder, for a longer time, with more focus than usual. It releases acetylcholine which calms down the ruminating mind and helps you to focus better.

Moreover, relaxing neurochemicals released by it, like serotonin and dopamine, further increase the focus and attention span for the work a person is doing.

This is highly beneficial for people whose jobs require plenty of concentration or are a monotonous type.

Be More Motivated

Kratom activates opioid receptors in the brain that make a person more motivated and energetic to complete the tasks. There is "adrenaline rush" that makes a person jump into action because noradrenaline and adrenaline are released that activate sympathetic nerves.

Besides this, it is also responsible for releasing serotonin and dopamine which boosts motivation. It helps a person to be motivated and focused yet serene and calm.

Improve Heart Health

Kratom leaves contain chemicals that are beneficial for the blood vessels, arteries, and hormones in the body. It also helps to reduce blood pressure.

This herb is very conducive for the heart, as it prevents a number of heart ailments by easing stress and tension. It helps to protect a person from health issues such as strokes, atherosclerosis, and heart attacks.

Sex Drive

It is used as a sexual enhancer and an aphrodisiac. It is very useful for the treatment of sexual disorders, such as low libido and erectile dysfunction.

Sleep Well

Kratom helps to regulate the sleep cycle. It can give relief to people who suffer due to parasomnia, insomnia, and night terrors. It enables a person to fall asleep more quickly and to have a deep and restorative sleep. This can in turn help in functioning better during the day. Sleep is sometimes underestimated as a factor for good health. Kratom can be helpful to improve sleep and contribute to overall well-being.

Reduce Inflammation

It has anti-inflammatory properties. Mitragynine, its basic active alkaloid, reduces inflammation. Kratom promotes healing. It reduces redness, swelling, and pain at the place of inflammation. Just like the pain relievers sold in the market, it has analgesic qualities.

Due to this, it is commonly used to give relief to patients who suffer from rheumatoid arthritis, osteoarthritis, and osteoporosis.

Combat Diarrhea

The nervous system (parasympathetic) influences a person's gastrointestinal tract. Kratom has the capacity to combat diarrhea, as it regulates this aspect of the nervous system. It slows down peristalsis.

It is a remarkable remedy of inflammatory diseases of the bowels, like ulcerative colitis and Crohn's disease, because of its anti-inflammatory properties.

Prevent Cancer

According to some researchers, Kratom can prevent cancer. It has similar effects like superoxide dismutase, glutathione, and natural antioxidants that prevent free radicals from forming in the body. This, in turn, lowers the risk for different types of cancer.

Lose Weight

Kratom has a mood enhancing and calming effect that is good for those who have a tendency to binge eat or have a sugar addiction. Besides this, it has the ability to regulate the satiety center located in the brain's hypothalamus. Therefore, a person who uses Kratom feels full quicker and eat less.

This is the reason why it is useful for people who do not want to put on excessive weight and remain healthy.

Fight Fatigue

Since ancient times, people have used Kratom to overcome symptoms of chronic fatigue. It promotes the circulation of blood and enhances the level of oxygen in the blood which boosts the metabolic processes and gives a lot of energy for at least 2-6 hours.

The neurochemicals released by it also provide energy, motivation, and focus that help to combat fatigue disorders and fatigue.

In the present, people are stressed and tired due to their busy lifestyle. Moreover, they do not get sufficient sleep. Kratom can help to alleviate this to some extent.

Studies Related to Kratom

Opiate Withdrawal Treatment

Zebrafish Case

According to Dr. Hassan and others, an experiment was done in 2007 in which 1.5 mg of morphine was given every day for two weeks to the zebrafish and they became addicted to it. When the morphine was stopped, they showed anxiety-related behaviors after 24 hours. Their erratic movements increased and they explored less. The level of their cortisol increased which shows that the withdrawal was stressful for them.

When mitragynine 2 mg was given to the fish the erratic behavior decreased and the cortisol levels also reduced.

Dr. Hassan and others concluded that Kratom is effective for treating the effects of opiate withdrawal.

Effect of Kratom on a Person's Mental Health

Drs. Zach Wolsh and Marc Swogger reviewed the relationship of Kratom to the mental health of human beings in 2017. They have confirmed that Kratom can be utilized as a means of harm reduction for those who suffer from opiate withdrawal.

Findings show that low doses of Kratom may be utilized as antidepressants and higher doses may have anxiolytic effects.

Kratom Stories

Kratom for Opioid Withdrawal

Kratom is getting increased acceptance as a treatment for opioid withdrawal symptoms. Here is a case of a person who used it to treat the chronic pain associated with withdrawal.

Description

One patient had abruptly stopped hydromorphone abuse. He self-managed the pain accompanied with the withdrawal by using Kratom. He ingested Kratom tea four times per day. He reported substantial relief from pain and improved alertness.

Kratom for Psoriatic Arthritis

A patient who had psoriatic arthritis and 2 ruptured discs used Kratom to get relief from the pain.

Description

A patient was undergoing treatment for these complaints when he had to move to another place. Consequently, he lost touch with his doctor who had been taking care of him. He suffered from pain and tried all sorts of pain killers which had no effect. After 6 months he learned about Kratom and his life changed altogether. It helped to alleviate the pain.

He says that Kratom is a plant which has countless medicinal uses. It is not some synthetic or chemical drug.

Kratom for Pain Relief

A patient who has Fibular Hemimelia and suffered from intense pain used Kratom to get rid of the pain.

Description

The patient did not have the major bones in his foot and ankle. It was excruciatingly painful to walk. He had to take medication for the pain throughout the day. After some time the doctor who was helping him retired and left him. He had to be on the waiting lists for doctors because no one wanted to take up his case.

He learned about Kratom and started using it. After that, he has been able to live a much better life.

Kratom Helped an Amputee to Overcome Addiction

An amputee suffered from constant pain and became a heavy opiate user. Kratom helped him to overcome the withdrawal symptoms.

Description

In order to combat pain, he started using opiates. He became an opiate addict. He realized that it was doing a lot of damage to his life. When he tried to stop using it, he suffered from withdrawal symptoms. Kratom helped him at that juncture and enabled him to start living a normal life.

Kratom for Lower Back Pain Relief

A lady who is very petite started having lower back problems after the birth of a child. Her pelvis and backbone started separating. It was very painful. Opiate drugs were administered for pain relief. They worked in the beginning but later they became ineffective. She started taking pain pills that made her feel horrible. At that time, she got to know about Kratom and used it. After that, she could get rid of the pain and live a much better life.

Side Effects and Toxicity

Even high doses of mitragynine show negligible toxicity. For instance, when rats were given Kratom's (leaf extract) 1000 mg oral doses or 806 mg isolated mitragynine there were no fatalities. When 9.2 milligrams mitragynine (IV) was injected in Rhesus monkeys they also had no fatalities.

However, this does not imply that Kratom is absolutely safe. The reason is that different quantities of adulterants and phytochemicals may be used in various preparations. Sufficient research has not been done in the field and the influence of regular use of Kratom for a long period of time, on a person's health is not known.

There has been a fivefold increase in seizures related to Kratom between the years 2005 to 2011 in Thailand.

Liver problems can occur after Kratom has been used regularly for 2 - 8 weeks. Symptoms include abdominal pain, jaundice, nausea, and dark urine.

There may be hyperpigmentation of cheeks in the people who consume a large quantity of Kratom because melanocytes are over stimulated.

Kratom may be cardiotoxic. But further research has to be done to confirm it.

Other issues associated with the use of Kratom include hypotension, sweating, erectile dysfunction, tremors, sleep problems, hair loss, anorexia, and dryness of the mouth.

Kratom should not be taken during pregnancy and breastfeeding. Besides causing some health issues the addiction may be carried over to the infants. However, there is limited evidence for it.

If Kratom is used regularly for more than a decade it may cause confusion, paranoid delusions, and hallucinations. Animal studies show that there is a connection between long term intake of Kratom and learning or memory problems.

Legality

In the US Kratom is considered to be one of the drugs of concern but it is not federally controlled. The plant has been banned in Wisconsin, Tennessee, Vermont, Alabama, Indiana, and Arkansas. Legislation is pending in other states.

It has been criminalized in the UK under the act related to psychoactive substances. Member states of the EU, including Poland, Sweden, and Denmark have taken various measures to control the use of the plant, as well as the active alkaloids found in it. The use of this plant is considered to be illegal in Malaysia, Australia, Thailand, Myanmar, and New Zealand.

Kratom has a legal status in Indonesia and it is exported globally. It had a legal status until 2003 in Malaysia. After that, it was included in the Poison Act. It was outlawed in Thailand in 1943. It belongs to the least dangerous substances category, that is Schedule 5 in the Narcotics Act of Thailand.

Countries in Europe where Kratom is Legal

- Austria

- Belgium
- Belarus
- Bulgaria
- Czech Republic
- Croatia
- Finland
- Denmark
- France
- Greece
- Germany
- Hungary
- Holland
- Netherlands
- Moldova
- Portugal
- Norway

Countries in Europe where Kratom is Illegal

- Ireland
- Latvia
- Italy
- Lithuania
- Romania
- Poland

- Sweden
- Russia
- United Kingdom
- Turkey

Future of Kratom

People have been keenly anticipating the future of Kratom. This opioid-like plant's fate has been uncertain for some time. Will it be made illegal? What are the regulations that will be imposed on it? Kratom users and scientists alike are concerned about it.

In 2017 the FDA submitted a recommendation to DEA for banning Kratom. Since then, researchers have been engaged in reviewing the recommendation.

Katherine Pfaff, DEA spokesperson, says that all the available data is being reviewed so that the final decision can be taken. But no time limit has been set for the decision, it could take months or even years.

A study of rats suggested that the drug could assist people to stop the consumption of opioids. It also showed that Kratom had a low potential for making people addicted to it. Addiction Biology contained a paper that showed mitragynine as well as 7-hydroxymitragynine, Kratom's two primary active molecules, have different effects. MG reduced the desire of the rats for morphine, the other molecule 7-HMG increased it. This indicated that the influence of Kratom might be more multifaceted and complex than scientists understood earlier. If Kratom is made illegal, both these molecules would be on an equal footing. This would make it very difficult for the researchers to explore Kratom and Kratom's components' therapeutic potential.

In case Kratom is put in the Schedule I, the highest degree of illegality, the scientists would need a special license from the DEA to conduct any study about it.

Walter Prozialeck, a pharmacology professor at Midwestern University analyzed 100 Kratom studies until 2016. Currently, he consults with Kratom researchers. According to him, unscientific reports show that compared to opioids, Kratom tends to be less addictive.

Prozialeck says, "By any measure, Kratom would be less harmful and less addictive than something like heroin. If you look at the evidence, you have to conclude that. But Kratom can induce a state of physical dependence."

Christopher McCurdy medicinal chemistry professor at Florida University says, "It is probably addictive, but its addictive equivalent is something like coffee, which isn't surprising because the leaf is in the coffee family."

His research done on mice supports the idea that Kratom can help to treat the symptoms of opioid withdrawal.

Supporters of Kratom say that it provides relief from depression, anxiety, and pain.

Dijon Evans, of Sacramento in CA, started using Kratom to get relief from chronic pain due to nerve damage. She says, "There was no high. I just felt better. I could move. I could breathe without all the pain. I felt alive again. I didn't feel buried by the pain."

This is the reason why some scientists are of the opinion that Kratom may have the potential to treat chronic pain as well as being an instrument to combat the addiction to various opioid medications.

The NIDA granted three and a half million dollars to McCurdy and colleagues for the purpose of studying the components of the plant in the next two years in order to understand how Kratom works and how it may be abused.

McCurdy says, "It's very clear that the National Institute on Drug Abuse wants to understand the science of this plant and the components of this plant because of the anecdotal stories and community of users showing this is working well to keep them off of opiates and the historical usage of this plant to wean people off opium or prescription drugs."

The DEA had made a move to ban Kratom in 2016 because it was considered to be a hazard for public safety. Due to public protest, it was not implemented. Those comments are being considered for the present scheduling decision.

The Kratom association of America submitted one petition from over forty thousand Americans in favor of Kratom. They issued a policy report, 27 pages long, saying that FDA had not provided the data to show that Kratom must be scheduled.

The association has been making efforts to encourage the manufacturers of Kratom to maintain the quality standards. McCurdy is working to bring together all the scientists from different parts of the world to participate in the 2nd international meeting related to Kratom research. The 1st was in Malaysia in 2017.

"The goal is to come together and share our work and determine where gaps are in the research that we need to collectively fill to gain a more solid scientific profile of the plant," he says. "But even though we are making advances on the science side, it is still a buyer-beware marketplace. I definitely believe there is legitimacy to using Kratom to self-treat opiate addiction. I believe it from the standpoint of the material we know is pure, unadulterated, and good. I just don't know if all products available are consistently pure and good; in other words, it is not clear that a product that is labeled Kratom is truly Kratom, in the traditional sense."

Kim DeMott, who was diagnosed with a number of diseases, was taking 28 medications per day, including a number of opioids, to get relief from chronic pain. Then she got to know about Kratom. She bought some online and made tea with it. She got relief with the very first cup. She has been trying to support the cause of Kratom.

DeMott says that the government's concerns regarding the quality are right. "I do agree that we should have some regulation. I support that because it is important to make sure companies follow good manufacturing processes and test their products," she says. "My hope is that we can all work together to find a way to keep it around and make sure everyone is getting something safe."

Therefore, instead of banning Kratom, it may be better to impose some regulations and implement some quality control measures to ensure that people get pure, unadulterated Kratom and the users can enjoy the real benefits that Kratom offers. So that Kratom can fulfill its purpose as an alternative remedy for various physical and mental ailments. At the same time, it can be an energizer, mood enhancer, and an asset for overall well-being.

Chapter V

How to Take Kratom

People chew fresh Kratom leaves after removing the central vein. Otherwise, they crush and powder them. They mix the powder with water or any other liquid and drink it. Some of them make a paste and consume it with water. While others take it in the form of capsules or extracts.

Kratom is sold in the market in the form of powder, capsules, and extracts. Each type has its own benefits and shortcomings. Let us see which form is most suitable for you.

Kratom Powder

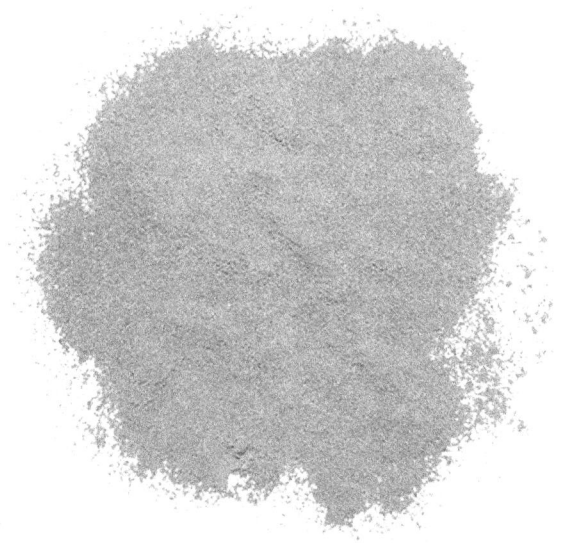

The Kratom leaves are dried and ground finely to make a powder. The harvesters and farmers pick the leaves of Kratom and then dry them outdoors or indoors. The method of processing depends on the vein type of Kratom.

Advantages of Powder

- This is the most common form in which Kratom is available. You can easily find the strand and vein type of your choice.
- It can be assimilated quickly by the body. Consequently, its effects can be experienced much faster compared to the other forms. Moreover, the result is more intense. You can feel when it "kicks in."
- The work of packaging the powder is simple for the manufacturers so it is cheaper than the capsule and extract forms of Kratom.
- The powder can be consumed in several ways. You can use it to make tea, or mix it in juice, smoothies, yogurt, applesauce, or water.

Disadvantages of Powder

- The powder tastes bitter and has a peculiar smell. It tastes somewhat like green tea that has been over-steeped or extremely strong matcha. Some people do not mind the taste but many people find it disgusting, horrible, and pungent.

- But all the powders may not be bitter. It depends on the vendors. Some of them sell certain powders which do not have a bad taste.
- When you swallow the powder it may stick to your tongue or throat and its bitter taste may linger for a long time. Or else, you may not feel very comfortable to swallow it.
- You have to measure and prepare the powder before consuming it. This makes it difficult to carry it with you to work or to the gym, or in case you have to spend time outdoors.
- You have to handle it carefully while measuring, otherwise you may spill the powder all over the place. If this happens you will lose some of the powder and will also have to waste time cleaning up.

Kratom Capsules

As Kratom is not very palatable and needs to be prepared, people have found better ways of consuming it. Therefore, vendors offer it in the form of capsules also.

Kratom capsules are available in five different sizes:

000 size - capsule has 1 g Kratom

00 size - capsule has 0.735 g Kratom

0 size - capsule has 0.5 g Kratom

1 size - capsule has 0.4 g Kratom

2 size - capsule has 0.3 g Kratom

Advantages of Capsules

- It is very convenient to take capsules. If you know the amount of Kratom in one capsule you can easily measure your dosage. Besides this, there are no chances of messing up the place, as is the case with the powder.
- It is easy to transport them. You can comfortably carry them with you when you go to work, or for a holiday, a hike, a day out in the city, and other similar occasions.
- It is easy to swallow the Kratom capsules. As there is a barrier in between the taste buds and the powder, you do not have to actually taste Kratom. This form is suitable for you if you dislike the taste of Kratom or are bothered by its smell.

Disadvantages of Capsules

- The capsules cost more than the powder. Extra time, manpower, and resources are needed to make them. As a result, the price of the capsules is high. Not many people manufacture these capsules.

- Every vendor may not sell Kratom capsules. All the varieties of Kratom may not be available in the form of capsules. Therefore, even if the seller has your choicest type of Kratoms, he may not sell it in the form of capsules.
- As the Kratom powder is inside the capsules the body takes a longer time to absorb them. So it may take a longer time to be effective. Some users have felt that the intensity of the results is also less.
- Mostly they make capsules with gelatin. If you take more capsules you consume more gelatin and other additives in the coating. This can upset the stomach.
- There may be some other chemicals in the coating of which you are not aware. You might be allergic to some of these substances. In order to avoid this, you should buy Kratom capsules from sellers whom you can trust.
- Kratom capsules might not be appropriate for vegans or vegetarians because of the material with which the coating is made. In case you are very particular about it, you can buy the powder of Kratom and make the capsules yourself by using some cellulose-based or vegetarian coating. This will be less expensive than buying the readymade ones.

Kratom Extract

This is the concentrated form of Kratom. Experts brew the powdered or crushed leaves for quite a long time to produce the extract. When almost all the water gets evaporated one thick paste is left that contains concentrated Kratom ingredients.

This paste may be further used to make a tincture, resin, oil, or concentrated powder.

The extracts are graded using a digit with an x, like 15x, 10x, or 1x. It indicates the amount of Kratom that has been used to make 1 g of the concentrate. For instance, 10x implies that 10 g of Kratom was reduced to make 1 g Kratom extract.

Advantages of Extract

- Since the extract is concentrated in small doses, it is more powerful. You can get the same results that you get with the powder by taking a relatively smaller dose of the extract.
- If you take the extract in the form of a liquid the body can absorb it quickly. So you can experience the results faster.
- The oil and tincture made from the Kratom extract can be used topically. For example, you can add Kratom to cosmetics, or make a body lotion at home, or make soap with it.

Disadvantages of Extract

- It is time-consuming and expensive to make Kratom extract. Moreover, the work has to be done by experts. So the price is much higher.
- Few users have found that the extracts are laced with other substances and opioids. So you should buy extracts only from credible and trustworthy vendors. You must check the contents before buying and see to it that you get the pure extract.
- Some users are of the opinion that tolerance to the extract develops faster than tolerance to the powder of Kratom.
- The extract's potency depends on the concentration of extract as well as the strain from which it originates. Due to this, it is difficult to determine the correct dose of the extract that should be taken. Consequently, there is more risk of taking an overdose of it.

Other Forms of Kratom

You can get Kratom in the form of crushed leaves as well. Although, this form is not very popular, some vendors sell this type of Kratom.

In Kratom powder, the veins and stems are removed. While in the form of crushed leaves all the parts are retained. As a result, the content is a little different. Some people feel that it is stronger than the powder.

However, you can consume this form of Kratom only by making tea with it. If you love tea then this could be the most suitable form for you.

The Ideal Way to Consume It

This may vary from one person to the other depending on each one's preferences and needs. But on the whole, Kratom powder is the best because it is easily available. It contains only pure Kratom and it is quite easy and simple to use it.

Methods of Preparation and Administration

Kratom Paste

You can consume it in the form of a paste with water.

Directions

- Put a single dose of Kratom powder in one cup.
- Put sufficient water to mix the powder and get a smooth paste.
- Mix well till the mixture becomes uniform.
- Fill a glass with water. Take a spoonful of the paste and swallow it. Drink some water. Again take some paste and drink water after swallowing it. In this way, you should take the complete dose. Do not swallow too much at a time and avoid choking.

Kratom Slurry

You can take the dose of Kratom in the form of a slurry.

Ingredients

- 7 g Kratom powder
- 1 cup water

Directions

- Put the Kratom powder in one cup of water.
- Stir well and swallow it quickly before the powder settles down in the cup. It may taste like a sour fibrous smoothie.
- Add some water to the cup, stir once and drink it so that if any powder is left on the sides you can consume that also.
- Take some fruit juice after that or mint flavored chewing gum to get rid of the slightly sour taste.

Note:

If you have some dried leaves which are whole, roughly crushed, or roughly ground you can put them in the coffee grinder or kitchen mixer and grind them at a high speed to form a powder.

Mix it with Food

You can mix Kratom with ice cream or applesauce. Its efficacy will not be affected if it is taken with food.

Toss and then Wash

In order to take Kratom in this way you have to put some powder in your mouth, then drink some liquid to swallow it. This method is very difficult because the dry powder may stick to the mouth or throat. You may blow out some of the powder from your mouth. If you resort to this method then take a small amount of powder at a time. Some people feel that this method helps to get the best effects of Kratom. But it is known that this method can cause constipation and other digestive issues.

Dosage

Measuring the Dosage

A good way to measure the dose is to use scales. Generally, Kratom doses contain some grams of the drug. You should use a scale that can correctly measure from one-tenth part of a gram to one gram. Plenty of scales that can measure correctly are available at affordable rates in the market You can buy and use one of them.

If you try to measure Kratom on the basis of volume, the result may not be as accurate as it is when you measure it by weight. This is because the volume may depend on how finely the substance has been ground. A teaspoon of finely powdered

Kratom weighs more than a teaspoon of leaves that have not been crushed finely or have been ground roughly.

A teaspoon of finely powdered Kratom sold in the market is about 2 grams and the extremely fine variety is 2.25 g. Three teaspoons are equal to one tablespoon. So one tablespoon of finely powdered Kratom is equal to six or seven grams.

One tablespoon is a medium size dosage of Kratom that has an average strength. It is a strong dose of high potency Kratom and a gentle dose of low potency Kratom.

A teaspoon of leaves that have been roughly ground weighs about 0.8 g.

Dosage

Actually, the dose of Kratom powder depends on each person's own experience. Every individual may get enjoyment from a different dosage. So the dosage has to be determined on the basis of personal trial.

After some time, a person may develop a tolerance for some particular strain so it is important to rotate the strains. Tolerance means that initially if 2 grams was the appropriate dosage after some time the person may find that 5 grams is more suitable and gives sufficient pleasure. An increase in tolerance is not considered to be good.

So some people are of the opinion that rotating the strains can avoid the development of tolerance. But there is no proof to confirm it. According to them every day you should consume a different strain and avoid taking similar strains for 3 consecutive days.

Hence while deciding the dosage you have to determine the correct quantity to be taken and how the strains have to be rotated.

Actually, the dose depends on a person's age, health status, and gender. Other factors, like the strain and the method of taking it, can also have an influence on the effect of Kratom. For example, the extract of Kratom is more potent compared to Kratom powder.

On the basis of a survey in which there were 8049 participants, it was found that taking 5 g of Kratom powder 3 times a day is adequate to get the desired results.

You should start with a small dose and increase the amount gradually until you get the effect that you want.

General Guidelines Regarding Dosage

Category - Low - moderate

Dose:

- 1 - 5 g of Kratom powder

Effects:

- Increased focus and energy
- Pain relief.

Category - High

Dose:

- 5 - 15 g of Kratom powder

Effects:

- Similar to opioid
- Sedation
- More risk of having side effects

Category - Risky

Dose:

- More than 15 g of Kratom powder

Effects:

- More risk of having serious side effects

Precautions

Before taking a new herb or treatment it is advisable to find out its potential risks. Even though Kratom has been used for ages, there is limited research to confirm its safety.

The side effects of this herb depend on the dose and the sensitivity level of the individual. Lower doses have stimulating effects which are positive for some users, while others may experience them in the form of agitation and anxiety.

Tremors, sweating, facial flushing, dizziness, vomiting, nausea, itching, and constipation are some other possible side effects of Kratom. However, serious effects like seizures are quite rare. They may occur when very high doses are consumed.

Besides this, Kratom can affect the capacity of the liver to metabolize some other medications and drugs. Therefore the people who are already taking some medication should seek professional advice before using Kratom.

Chapter VI

What to Buy

You must buy good quality Kratom from a trustworthy vendor. For this, you should do thorough research before buying Kratom. You can read reviews about various vendors on the internet or talk to qualified people who have knowledge about Kratom. You can also get some tips from the users of Kratom.

There many online sellers of Kratom who sell it in the form of dried leaves, or its extracts. It is also sold in the form of powder and capsules. But you should be cautious and check the brand and labels. Sometimes they may sell fake Kratom, sell some other herb in the name of Kratom, or mix Kratom with some other herb or chemical.

Buy from Shops

Kratom products are available in various head shops and small stores. They are sold in the form of bags of powdered leaves, or as packages of capsules. Sometimes the capsules contain powdered leaves and are just enough for small doses. Even if they contain Kratom extract, the extract is very weak and all the capsules have to be taken before you can see any effects. Their prices start from $20 onwards.

Purchase Online

The quality of Kratom sold in the stores is inconsistent and very expensive. So it is advisable to find some reputed online seller who can provide good quality Kratom at reasonable prices.

The online vendors have to keep up with the competition in the field. There are a number of forums which review and rate the quality of their goods. They have to build a reputation for selling high-quality goods if they want a wide customer base. So their goods are better than those sold in the head shops and stores.

Brands of Kratom

Some of the most popular brands of Kratom are:

- Krave Kratom
- Club 13
- Bumble Bee
- O.P.M.S.
- Blue Magic
- Klarity Kratom

These brands sell Kratom that is worth millions every year. They provide Kratom products in the form of extracts, capsules, and powders.

Krave Kratom

Krave Kratom has been selling Kratom for more than 6 years. It offers 6 varieties of Kratom. They are:

- Maeng Da
- White Thai
- Bali
- Green Malay
- Trainwreck
- CBD Infused
- Gold
- Red Vein

Each strain is available in the form of capsules. There are 5 sizes of bottles that contain 500, 300, 150, 75, and 30 capsules each.

The powder is available in 3 sizes of 250 g, 120 g, and 60 g.

Bumble Bee

Bumble Bee offers 6 varieties of Kratom. They are:

- Maeng Da (Premium)
- Bali Gold
- Green Borneo
- White Borneo
- Red Borneo
- Hello Vietnam

The strains are available in the form of capsules in bottles of 500, 300, 90, and 40 capsules each.

The powder is sold in 3 sizes of 250 g, 120 g, and 60 g.

Club 13

Club 13 has been selling Kratom since 1999.

They provide these powders:

- Bali Red
- Green Malay
- Indo White
- Connoisseur Blend
- Maeng Da - Green, Red, White

The powders are available in 1 pound, 150 g, 90 g, 30 g, and 15 g sizes.

These strains are sold in the form of capsules in bottles containing 120, 50, 25, and 10 capsules each.

O.P.M.S.

O.P.M.S. has a long standing in the industry. The products that they offer are:

- Silver line is available in the form of capsules in bottles containing 60, 30, and 16 capsules each.
- Blister packs come in boxes containing 64 and 32 capsules.
- The powders are available in 28 g packages.
- Gold line is available in packages of 5, 3, and 2 capsules (extra strength capsules) packages.
- Silver Thai, Malay, and Malay Special, and Maeng Da strains are available.
- The company offers 8 ml extract of Kratom that is very popular and powerful.

Buying Different Strands

Some people, who have the opinion that rotating the strands can prevent the development of tolerance, suggest that every new user should buy four to seven one-ounce Kratom bags. Each bag must have different strains of different colors of Kratom.

For example:

- One-ounce bag containing Green Malay
- One-ounce bag containing Red Bali
- One-ounce bag containing White Bali
- One-ounce bag containing Yellow Vietnam
- One-ounce bag containing Wild Green. (Premium)

The first dose can be of Red Bali, the second could be a mixture of Wild Green and White Bali.

You can mix up the Kratom dose to get the benefit or enjoyment that you desire.

This is the method of taking powdered Kratom.

Kratom Recipes

Chocolate Milkshake with Kratom

Taking Kratom in this form is very suitable because the bitter flavor is masked by chocolate milk.

Ingredients

- 1 cup almond milk (chocolate flavored)
- 1 dose of Kratom powder

Directions

- Put one dose of Kratom powder in a glass.
- Then put the same amount of milk, probably two tablespoons of milk.
- Mix well so that a smooth paste is formed. If there are any lumps add some more milk and stir.
- Add the rest of the milk and mix well.

Kratom Tea

You can use this recipe to make tea for eight strong doses of Kratom.

Ingredients

- 2 oz Kratom leaves (dried and crushed)
- 4 cups of water

Directions

- Put the leaves along with the water in one pot.
- Simmer the contents for 15 minutes.
- Pour the liquid through a strainer into a bowl and store it.
- Put another four cups of water in the pot. Put the leaves back in it. Repeat the previous steps. Discard the leaves after straining the liquid.
- Then put all the liquid together and boil once again in the pot till the quantity is reduced to one cup.

You can mix black tea or any herbal tea with this tea to get a better flavor. You can even add some sugar or honey and sweeten it.

You can keep this tea in the fridge for 5 days. If you want to store it for a longer period you should add some alcohol to preserve it.

Chapter VII

Frequently Asked Questions

1. Can Kratom be detected through drug tests?

Kratom cannot be detected through the standard type or the enhanced type of drug tests. Even though it is similar to opiates it is less likely for it to trigger false positives.

Specialized laboratory tests like GC-MS can detect it in urine. However, these tests are not usually conducted.

Kratom contains alkaloids which bind with the opiate receptors but structurally they are not related to opiate drugs. Therefore it is not detected.

Technically, the alkaloids can be detected in the body fluids. But normally such a test is not done.

2. Can the herb bring about psychological trauma?

There could be some connection between prolonged and regular use of Kratom (or addiction to it) and the occurrence of deluded thoughts. But moderate use is less likely to cause any psychological problems.

The "high" brought about by Kratom is quite manageable and mild compared to other kinds of psychoactive substances.

3. Does it have any risks?

Mostly Kratom is quite safe for healthy individuals. But it is always better to begin with a very small test dose so that you can know whether it is suitable for you or not.

It may pose a risk for people whose liver is damaged. Effects on pregnant women are not known. But there are chances of transmitting the addiction to the babies.

4. Is it permitted to grow Kratom at home?

This depends on the law of the state where you live. But it may be permitted to grow it for aesthetic reasons even if it is banned in the state.

5. Which is the safest method of taking Kratom?

Most people take it orally, using the toss and wash method or mixing it in a drink. You can add it to food items such as yogurt, fruit juice, chocolate milk, or applesauce to mask the taste. Otherwise, you can take it in the form of capsules.

Smoking Kratom is not advisable because a large number of leaves are needed for this purpose. It is necessary to brew, filter, and evaporate the dried Kratom before smoking it. After this process, it forms into a syrupy resin. This is added to the leaves of palas palm, in one long "madat" pipe's bowl.

Chewing the fresh leaves of Kratom is also feasible. The veins and ribs should be taken out before chewing. You can get the effects by chewing half of one eight-inch leaf. But people generally chew one to three leaves.

Kratom is also available in the form of extracts and tinctures. But these may contain some other ingredients as well.

6. What is the difference between strains?

All the strains contain similar active alkaloids. But their potency may vary substantially from one another.

7. Can Kratom be used to microdose?

This substance is not appropriate for microdosing as there is a likelihood of damaging the liver. Moreover, it is not clearly known whether it is active at the sub-perceptual dosage.

8. Does Kratom produce tolerance?

Tolerance builds up if it is used frequently, that is more than one or two times a week. Abstinence may be required for several weeks to get back the normal sensitivity. Besides this, there is cross-tolerance influence with morphine.

9. Is it possible to mix Kratom with some other drugs?

It is not advisable to mix Kratom with other drugs because most of the cases of Kratom users who suffered from seizures or death involved other drugs being used in combination with Kratom.

It should not be taken along with stimulants like cocaine, an excessive quantity of caffeine, yohimbine, and amphetamines. It must not be combined with depressants like opiates, alcohol, and benzodiazepines.

Some antidepressants and MAOIs, like ayahuasca, should be avoided.

10. What are the substances with which Kratom can be combined?

Combining Kratom with certain substances has been reported to be safe and have pleasant effects. Kratom and ordinary tea can be combined without any risk. People use it with tea made of poppy flowers. Red poppy itself has a mild narcotic influence. They use it with tea made of blue lotus. The tea prepared in this manner is sedating and euphoriant.

Some of them combine it with a small quantity of alcohol. Large quantities should not be used. There are people who enjoy smoking cannabis or tobacco when they are under Kratom's influence. However, while doing this it is necessary to be careful and not to fall asleep and drop the lit smoking items near yourself.

11. How long does the effect of Kratom last?

Usually, the effects last for about five to six hours. The effects are felt after thirty to forty minutes of ingestion, if it is taken on an empty stomach. The effects may be seen after sixty to ninety minutes, if it is taken when there is some food in the stomach. It may take a little longer to see the effects if it is taken in the form of capsules because they may take some time to dissolve.

12. What are the things that should not be done after taking Kratom?

After taking Kratom you should not engage in any hazardous activity as you may fall asleep. You should not drive when you are under Kratom's influence. Do not do it even when you are feeling stimulated, instead of feeling sleepy, because sleepiness might come without warning. You should not climb ladders or work with power tools after taking Kratom. Do not fall asleep after placing a pan on the stove. Be careful and use your common sense.

13. Is it habit forming?

If Kratom is taken responsibly, it may not be habit forming. In case it is taken occasionally like a recreational drug there is no chance of dependency. If it is taken every day for a long time it may turn into a habit that is difficult to break. Just like tobacco, coffee, or alcohol it may become a daily habit. Therefore, it is important to set some usage guidelines and limits for yourself.

However, people who use it to overcome an opiate addiction might have to take it every day to avoid the symptoms of opiate withdrawal. Those who have chronic pain may need to take it regularly.

Interestingly, studies show that opiate drugs rarely tend to be addictive. The same is applicable to Kratom because its action is similar to them.

14. What are the guidelines for safe usage of Kratom?

It is better to be cautious and safe. Therefore it is recommended that people should use Kratom only one or two times a week. It is even better to take it just one or two times a month. That means Kratom must be kept as an occasional special treat. By doing this you will get greater pleasure when you use it and you will not become dependent on it.

15. Can it cause overdoses?

Unlike other opioids, Kratom does not lead to respiratory depression. So there is less likelihood of a fatal overdose. Drs. Oliver Grundmann and Henningfield say that most of the Kratom related issues for which people call at the centers for poison control have a minor to moderate severity. The user surveys conducted by Dr. Henningfield show that less than 1% of the respondents sought mental health or medical treatment associated with Kratom consumption.

16. Have any health problems been reported due to the use of Kratom?

There is less likelihood of having health problems unless a person consumes a large quantity of Kratom on a daily basis. The people who consume it every day and are dependent on Kratom may lose weight, their face may have dark pigmentation, and they may experience withdrawal symptoms when they quit suddenly. They may suffer muscle pain, irritability, runny nose, jerking of the muscles, and diarrhea.

There are fewer chances of health problems in users who take Kratom occasionally. Like any medicine or drug, the reactions may vary. Some people may have some allergic or unusual reaction even after using it responsibly.

17. What are the active constituents in Kratom?

Several tryptamine alkaloids are present in Kratom. Out of them mitragynine, as well as 7-hydroxymitragynine, are the most important. They are mainly responsible for the pain-relieving, stimulating, euphoric, and sedative effects of Kratom. The structure of these alkaloids is similar to yohimbine but their effects are different from it.

18. How to grow Kratom?

It is possible to grow Kratom as a house plant. But as it grows to be quite large, it needs to be cut. It grows well in humid environments. It does not like cold weather. The plant cannot tolerate frost.

In places which have a temperate climate, you can grow potted plants outdoors when the weather is quite warm and grow them indoors at other times. In places where there is a tropical climate, the plants can be grown outdoors throughout the year.

Plants can be grown from cuttings. When the plants are actively growing, they need to be fertilized lightly at intervals of a few weeks.

19. What effects does Kratom have?

Kratom is one unique herbal drug. Its moderate dose is stimulating and a higher dose has a sedating effect. This is because active alkaloids present in Kratom have stimulant as well as sedative effects. Which one predominates depends on the dosage and the sensitivity of the person using it.

As a stimulant, it makes the mind more alert, increases physical energy, sexual energy, motivation, and the ability to perform strenuous and monotonous physical tasks. It elevates the mood and the person becomes more friendly, talkative, and sociable.

The stimulating effect of Kratom is different from the CNS stimulants like amphetamine drugs or caffeine. It is a cognitive stimulant rather than a physical stimulant.

As a sedative, analgesic, and euphoric it makes the person less sensitive towards emotional or physical pain. It gives a sense of calmness and pleasure.

You may find music more enjoyable. In such a state if you make your room semi-dark, lie down and close your eyes, and listen to some favorite music you may enjoy a delightful state that can be described as 'waking-dreaming' when you will be in a dreamy reverie.

Sometimes a person may experience sweating and itching. The pupils may become constricted. You might feel nauseated. At such a time you should relax and lie down. The nausea will subside quickly.

20. Are any Kratom products adulterated?

Sometimes chemical analysis of certain Kratom products shows that they are mixed with some other substances. Some sellers do this to decrease the cost and get higher profits. Otherwise, they do it to increase the effects by mixing synthetic drugs.

It has been found that certain items labeled as Kratom products contain O-desmethyltramadol, a "designer drug" that is a very dangerous opioid drug.

Analysis has shown that Kratom has been laced with morphine and hydrocodone in some cases. These opioids may have effects similar to Kratom but their effects are more dangerous.

Therefore, it is essential to buy Kratom products from trustworthy sources where they are routinely tested and then sold. On its own Kratom is quite safe. But unscrupulous vendors are making its consumption dangerous by acting in a reckless manner and selling adulterated goods.

Final Thoughts

Pros and Cons of Kratom

Kratom is a wonderful herb that has many medicinal uses. Its advantages outweigh its disadvantages. Actually, Kratom is very beneficial for the mind as well as the body, if it is taken in the right quantity. It can cause harm only if it is taken excessively and in large quantities.

Advantages

Energy Booster: You can add a few chopped leaves of Kratom to your tea and feel refreshed and enthused. It elevates the heart rate. It has a calming effect and reduces restlessness. Studies show that it gives an overall boost to your energy and helps you to focus on your work.

Mood Enhancer: It gives a boost to your mood and uplifts your feelings. It makes you feel euphoric, happy, and satisfied. Kratom has a miraculous effect on the mind and makes it peaceful. It helps to remove negative emotions.

Improves Concentration: It dispels brain fog and helps to concentrate on studies and work.

Stress Reliever: Kratom fights with anxiety and stress. It works as a sedative and calms the mind. It helps to ease nervousness and tension.

Pain Reliever: It helps in relieving pain due to various reasons. It assists in curing infections and diseases. It is used to treat intestinal infections, diarrhea, muscle pain, and cough.

Besides this, most of the people who have used Kratom say that it is useful for treating restless legs disorder, arthritis, and fibromyalgia.

Disadvantages of Kratom

It can cause:

- Insomnia
- Frequent urination
- Weight loss
- Nausea
- Vomiting
- Excessive sweating
- Darkening of the skin
- Aggressive behavior
- Depression
- Paranoia
- Constant craving for drugs

The herb has given rise to controversy because some people argue that it is useful to overcome the withdrawal symptoms of pain pills and opiates like heroin. However, the patients use it without consulting any licensed health personnel and without any dependable instructions. The dangers and latent side effects of the product and its interactions with the other drugs are not given due consideration

Another reason is that at present the DEA has not scheduled Kratom. The decision to schedule it was almost taken but it was stalled because of public resistance to it. Those who are in favor of the herb argue that other alternatives for pain medications should be provided before scheduling Kratom.

Moreover, there are no regulations for the herb that is claimed to be safe by its proponents. Consequently, it is sometimes adulterated and sold by the vendors. The substances mixed with them can make its consumption hazardous.

Conclusion

Low doses of Kratom have been used to improve productivity and keep fatigue at bay. Moderate doses have been used to treat pain, diarrhea, cough, and opioid withdrawal symptoms.

In recent times, it has also become popular for recreational purposes in the western countries to lift the mood and enhance physical performance. It is also used for its euphoric effects.

A review of the literature available in the medical databases shows that users have reported its sedative and stimulatory effects. Its positive influence in managing pain, and inflammation, and in supporting immunity as well as the health of the blood vessels is also documented.

Ninety-five articles about the use of Kratom in both western and eastern countries were analyzed. Subjective benefits were experienced by the users. The reports from the traditional users of Kratom in Southeast Asia showed that they felt happy, mentally calm, strong, and active. The users in the western countries said that they had more physical energy, were more alert, there was more sexual arousal, and they experienced euphoria, and greater empathy. The users who took higher doses said that it relieved the pain and had sedative effects. It made the physical and emotional pain dull.

Now that you know about this wonderful herb you can easily get rid of your aches and other health problems. You can give a boost to your body and mind. Above all, you can improve your quality of life by using the correct amount of this amazing gift of nature.

Bibliography

1. Aaron. (2018, January 12). The pros and cons of Kratom. Retrieved from

https://www.narcononnewliferetreat.org/blog/the-pros-and-cons-of-Kratom.html

2. Benefits of Kratom. Retrieved from

https://therenegadepharmacist.com/benefits-of-Kratom/

3. Boyer, E.W. Self-treatment of opioid withdrawal using Kratom. Retrieved from

https://www.ncbi.nlm.nih.gov/pmc/articles/PMC3670991/#S5title

4. Clopton, J. (2019, February 11). Regulations are on hold as Kratom debate rages. Retrieved from

https://www.webmd.com/mental-health/addiction/news/20190211/regulations-

are-on-hold-as-Kratom-debate-rages

5. Hess, P. (2018, November 19). Federal authorities tight-lipped on when Kratom's future will be revealed. Retrieved from

https://www.inverse.com/article/50958-will-Kratom-be-made-illegal-soon

6. Jerry. (2019, May 17). Kratom user's guide & dosage tips. Retrieved from

https://Kratommasters.com/Kratom-dosage-tips-for-new-users/

7. Kratom regions. (2018, July 12). Retrieved from

http://Kratomtimes.com/Kratom-regions/

8. Kratom strains and their different colors, red, white or green? Retrieved from

https://www.Kratomgardens.com/en/Kratom-strains

9. Kroll, D. (2016, September 30). The benefits of Kratom, and risks of Kratom extracts, from the people who use the botanical medicine. Retrieved from

https://www.forbes.com/sites/davidkroll/2016/09/30/the-benefits-of-Kratom-

from-the-people-who-use-the-botanical-medicine/#7e1b95de9ab0

10. McGuinness, E. (n.d.). Do the benefits of Kratom outweigh the risks? Retrieved from

https://www.daimanuel.com/2018/07/04/do-the-benefits-of-Kratom-outweigh-the-risks/

11. My Kratom Club. (2019, March 15). Best Kratom brands - How to find your brand. Retrieved from

https://myKratomclub.com/best-Kratom-brands/

12. Pros and cons of Kratom. (2018, September 12). Retrieved from

http://www.dolansrestaurant.com/2018/09/12/pros-and-cons-of-Kratom/

13. Siebert, D. (2016, October 12). The Kratom user's guide. Retrieved from

http://www.sagewisdom.org/Kratomguide.html

14. Speciosa Guide. (2018, September 21). Best way to take Kratom: Powder, capsules, or extract. Retrieved from

https://speciosaguide.com/best-way-take-Kratom-powder-capsules-extract/

15. Strains, effects, and dosage. Retrieved from

https://www.Kratomscience.com/strains-effects-and-dosage/

16. The beginner's guide to Kratom. Retrieved from

https://www.Kratomscience.eu/the-beginners-guide-to-Kratom/

17. The essential guide to Kratom. Retrieved from

https://thethirdwave.co/psychedelics/Kratom/

18. Vandergriendt, C. (2018, December 19). Can you use Kratom for depression and anxiety? Retrieved from

https://www.healthline.com/health/depression/Kratom-for-depression#types

19. Where to buy Kratom. Retrieved from

https://www.Kratomscience.com/buy-Kratom/

20. Where to buy Kratom. Retrieved from

https://www.Kratomscience.eu/where-to-buy-Kratom/